Protecting, promoting and supporting breast-feeding: the special role of maternit

A Joint WHO/UNICEF Statement

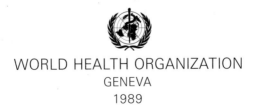

WORLD HEALTH ORGANIZATION

GENEVA

1989

Reprinted 1990, 1991, 1994

ISBN 92 4 156130 0
© World Health Organization 1989

PRINTED IN SWITZERLAND
89/7942 — 90/8399 — 91/8918 — 72500
94/10017 — Gloor-Luder SA — 5000

Contents

Ten steps
to successful breast-feeding

Every facility providing maternity services and care for newborn infants should:

1. Have a written breast-feeding policy that is routinely communicated to all health care staff.

2. Train all health care staff in skills necessary to implement this policy.

3. Inform all pregnant women about the benefits and management of breast-feeding.

4. Help mothers initiate breast-feeding within a half-hour of birth.

5. Show mothers how to breast-feed, and how to maintain lactation even if they should be separated from their infants.

6. Give newborn infants no food or drink other than breast milk, unless *medically* indicated.

7. Practise rooming-in — allow mothers and infants to remain together — 24 hours a day.

8. Encourage breast-feeding on demand.

9. Give no artificial teats or pacifiers (also called dummies or soothers) to breast-feeding infants.

10. Foster the establishment of breast-feeding support groups and refer mothers to them on discharge from the hospital or clinic.

Foreword

In our world of diversity and contrast, we believe that this statement on the role of maternity services in promoting breast-feeding is striking for its universal relevance. The principles affirmed here apply *anywhere* maternity services are offered, irrespective of such labels as "developed" and "developing", "North" and "South", "modern" and "traditional". And the health professionals and other workers responsible for these services are well placed to apply them by providing the leadership needed to sustain, or if necessary re-establish, a "breast-feeding culture".

While discoveries are still being made about the many benefits of breast milk and breast-feeding, few today would openly contest the maxim "breast is best". Yet slogans, however accurate, are no substitute for action. That is why we invite all those concerned with providing maternity services to study this statement to see how they are helping or hindering breast-feeding. Are they encouraging and supporting mothers in every possible way? We urge them, wherever they might be, to ensure that their services are fully mobilized to this end and thereby to bear witness to the unequalled excellence of breast-feeding for infants and mothers alike.

Hiroshi Nakajima, M.D., Ph.D.
Director-General
World Health Organization

James P. Grant
Executive Director
United Nations Children's Fund

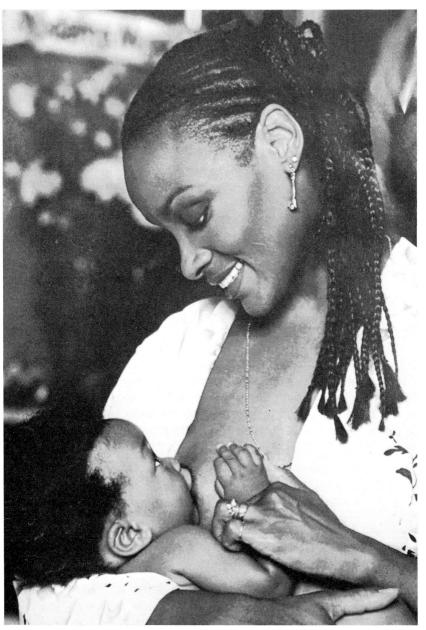

WHO/PAHO (19834)

1. Introduction

Breast-feeding is an unequalled way of providing ideal food for the healthy growth and development of infants and has a unique biological and emotional influence on the health of both mother and child. The anti-infective properties of breast milk help to protect infants against disease and there is an important relation between breast-feeding and child-spacing. For these reasons, professional and other health workers serving in health care facilities should make every effort to protect, promote and support breast-feeding, and to provide expectant and new mothers with objective and consistent advice in this regard.

The prevalence and duration of breast-feeding have declined in many parts of the world for a variety of social, economic and cultural reasons. With the introduction of modern technologies and the adoption of new life-styles, the importance attached to this traditional practice has been noticeably reduced in many societies. However unwittingly, health services frequently contribute to this decline, either by failing to support and encourage mothers to breast-feed or by introducing routines and procedures that interfere with the normal initiation and establishment of breast-feeding. Common examples of the latter are separating mothers from their infants at birth, giving infants glucose water by bottle and teat before lactation has been initiated, and routinely encouraging the use of breast-milk substitutes.

For breast-feeding to be successfully initiated and established, mothers need the active support, during pregnancy and following birth, not only of their families and communities but also of the entire health system. Ideally, all health workers with whom expectant and new mothers come into contact will be committed to promoting breast-feeding, and will be able to provide appropriate information as well as demonstrate a thorough practical knowledge of breast-feeding management.

Too often, however, the reality is quite different: health personnel may have insufficient knowledge about breast-feeding and little experience in providing appropriate support for mothers, and may be unaware of the main factors that determine whether or not mothers breast-feed and for how long. Their training has frequently oriented them more towards bottle-feeding, as a "modern technology" that can be taught and supervised, than towards preparing mothers for successful breast-feeding, which they may regard as old-fashioned and no longer warranting particular attention. Not surprisingly, they may also be ignorant of the negative impact that accepted hospital routines and procedures (often established on grounds of efficiency or resource constraints, or for supposed scientific reasons) can have on the successful initiation and establishment of breast-feeding. Impediments to breast-feeding initiation range from the physical layout of maternity wards and hospitals and the organization of their services to the attitudes of doctors, nurses, administrators and other staff.

WHO and UNICEF believe that, of the many factors that affect the normal initiation and establishment of breast-feeding, health care practices, particularly those related to the care of mothers and newborn infants, stand out as one of the most promising means of increasing the prevalence and duration of breast-feeding. Reasons for this include the predisposition of health workers to promote health-enhancing behaviour, the very nature and function of health care facilities, and the fact that, apart from good will, few additional resources are required to maintain or introduce appropriate routines and procedures.

For this reason, WHO and UNICEF wish to encourage a review of how health services promote or hinder breast-feeding, so that policies, practices and routines that enhance its early initiation and establishment may be reinforced and those that interfere with it may be modified. The present statement concentrates on the relatively brief period of prenatal, delivery and perinatal care provided in maternity wards and clinics, which is critical for the successful initiation and maintenance of breast-feeding. This is when interaction between health personnel and mothers is closest and where health care routines have the greatest influence on mothers' attitudes towards breast-feeding and perceptions about their ability to breast-feed. The statement and its annex can serve as a check-list of the main actions that should be taken by and through maternity services to ensure that breast-feeding is effectively promoted and facilitated.

The statement is addressed to the competent authorities in countries — health and nutrition policy-makers; managers of maternal and child health and family planning services; clinicians, midwives, nursing personnel and other support staff in maternity services and facilities for the care of newborn infants; health workers' organizations; and mothers' support groups. Its purpose is twofold: to increase awareness of the critical role that health services play in protecting and promoting breast-feeding, and to describe what should be done to provide mothers with appropriate information and support. The focus is on the types of actions to be taken rather than on details of their content, for example the structure of messages or means for delivering them. Such specifics are best decided on according to local circumstances. Readers are thus invited to adapt the statement and to use it to determine how best to organize their maternity services so as to promote and facilitate the initiation and establishment of breast-feeding by the mothers in their care.

Suggested action

Institutions and programmes providing maternity services and care for newborn infants should review their policies and practices relating to breast-feeding. If they have not already done so, they should develop breast-feeding policy guidelines covering care for expectant and new mothers and newborn infants, and relevant information, education and training. They should ensure that these guidelines are communicated to all staff concerned, and should undertake periodically to evaluate their effectiveness.

2. Preparing health workers to promote and support breast-feeding

Essential messages about breast-feeding

A number of essential messages about breast-feeding should be communicated to all health workers. They serve as a basis for understanding the relation between health services and the successful initiation and establishment of breast-feeding, and the role that health care facilities should play in protecting, promoting and supporting it. These messages include:

- Breast-feeding is an unequalled way of providing ideal food for the healthy growth and development of all normal infants. Ideally, exclusive breast-feeding will be the norm for the first 4–6 months of life.
- Virtually all women can lactate; genuine physiopathological reasons for not being able to breast-feed are rare.
- Anxiety associated with unfounded fears of lactation failure (the inability to produce milk) and of milk insufficiency (the inadequacy of breast milk for meeting the nutritional needs of the normal infant) is one of the most common reasons for mothers' failing to initiate breast-feeding, interrupting it prematurely, or beginning complementary feeding before it is nutritionally required. Emotional support will strengthen a mother's confidence that she can successfully breast-feed.
- Anaesthesia, strong sedation, prolonged labour, surgical intervention, and other sources of stress, discomfort and fatigue for mothers and infants impede the initiation of lactation.
- Close mother–child contact immediately following birth and frequent sucking at the breast are the best stimulus for milk secretion.
- The correct positioning of the infant at the breast is important to facilitate feeding, ensure milk supply and help prevent sore or cracked nipples and breast engorgement.

- The first milk — colostrum — is of particular nutritional and health value to the infant given its high content of proteins and fat-soluble vitamins and its anti-infective properties. It is the infant's first immunization.
- Under normal circumstances the neonate requires no water or other food whatsoever during the first 2–4 days after birth while lactation is being initiated.
- Giving any other food or drink to the breast-fed infant before about 4 months of age is usually unnecessary and may entail

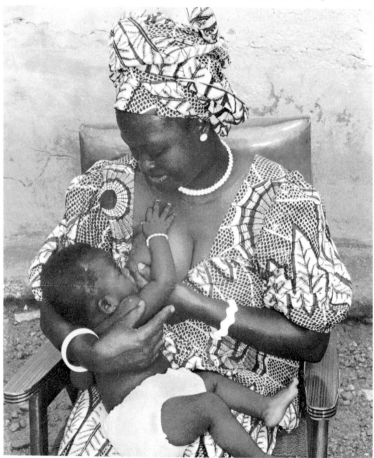

WHO/I.K. Oduro
(entry in the International Photo Competition "Health for all — all for health")

risks, for example making the infant more vulnerable to diarrhoeal and other diseases. Because of its effect on sucking and milk secretion, any other food or drink given before complementary feeding is nutritionally required may interfere with the initiation or maintenance of breast-feeding.

> **Suggested action**
>
> Institutions and programmes providing maternity services and care for newborn infants should ensure that essential messages about breast-feeding are communicated to all staff concerned.

Training health workers

Staff training merits particular attention, especially for health workers directly responsible for caring for mothers and providing them with objective and consistent information on appropriate infant feeding. Health workers should not only be knowledgeable about the health, nutritional and physiological aspects of appropriate feeding; they should also be familiar with the mechanics of breast-feeding, its various psychosocial influences, and possible difficulties and how to overcome them. Knowledge alone is insufficient, of course; staff also need a positive attitude towards breast-feeding, which comes with experience and an understanding of the many incomparable advantages that this feeding mode offers mothers and infants alike.

> **Suggested action**
>
> The staff of maternity wards and clinics for maternal and child health and family planning should receive appropriate basic and in-service training on the health benefits of breast-feeding and on lactation management. All other health workers should be made fully aware of the importance of breast-feeding.

3. Where and when health workers should act

The critical role health workers play in protecting, promoting and supporting breast-feeding should be seen in the context of their broad social commitment. As authorities on appropriate infant nutrition and health care, they are in a unique position to influence the organization and functioning of health services provided to mothers before, during and after pregnancy and delivery.

The broad social context of action by health workers

Promoting and facilitating breast-feeding is not the sole responsibility of the health services nor of any single health programme or category of health worker. Ideally, it will be viewed as one of a number of important health and nutrition policies that merits encouragement by everyone in society. The support to breast-feeding provided by health care services, sustained by the knowledge, skills and commitment of health workers, will then be part of society's commitment to appropriate feeding practices for infants and young children.

Women's experience and education, from earliest childhood, will influence their attitudes and performance in relation to breast-feeding later in life. Regularly seeing other women breast-feed, especially in the same family or social group, is thus one of a number of important ways in which girls and young women can develop positive attitudes towards breast-feeding.

Where a "bottle-feeding culture" prevails, girls and young women are typically deprived of positive role models of breast-feeding in their everyday experience. Not surprisingly, adult women in this environment frequently have little or no information about breast-feeding; have little or no experience with its mechanics; lack confidence about their ability to breast-feed; and have no close family member, friend or other means of social support to aid them in overcoming problems they may encounter in initiating breast-feeding. In extreme cases, whole generations of young mothers have never seen a woman breast-feed and know nothing about a practice that they consider old-fashioned and no longer necessary. It is clearly preferable not to wait until these women are attending prenatal clinics or are in maternity wards giving birth before trying to educate them about breast-feeding and motivate them to breast-feed their own infants. Even if the will is there, few mothers are likely to succeed under such circumstances.

Girls from early childhood and on into adolescence should be positively oriented towards breast-feeding through both their life experience and formal education. Breast-feeding mothers should be encouraged to let children of all ages, but particularly girls, observe how they feed and care for their infants. The advantages of breast-feeding should be emphasized in the context of family-life education for adolescents, and complete information should be given about the important relation between breast-feeding and child-spacing.

The key is to prevent a self-perpetuating cycle of ignorance about breast-feeding from taking hold, particularly in societies that are experiencing the dislocations associated with rapid modernization, or, where such a cycle has been established, to break it through broad, intensive and sustained educational efforts. Health workers should lead in preserving or re-establishing a "breast-feeding culture" by promoting a positive attitude towards breast-feeding in society as a whole, and stimulating and working closely with community leaders to achieve this end. The role model provided by female health workers who breast-feed their infants is one important means, while providing these women with the time and facilities to breast-feed is an active indication of broad societal support on their behalf.

Structure and functioning of health services

There are many aspects of the structure and functioning of health services that will either facilitate or interfere with what health personnel can do to protect, promote and support breast-feeding. Often, procedures and routines are introduced for seemingly valid scientific and organizational reasons, or for the convenience of the health care staff in providing what are perceived as efficient and effective services. Rarely, however, is thought given to the implications of these procedures and routines for breast-feeding practice. The significance, in this context, of whether mothers and infants remain together after delivery (a practice commonly referred to as "rooming-in") and of certain neonatal care routines is discussed on pages 20–22.

The attitudes prevailing in a health service are also important for breast-feeding. For example, staff can have a positive influence by demonstrating to a mother and her family that they consider pregnancy, delivery and breast-feeding a positive experience that should take place in a hospitable and supportive environment. In addition, many procedures and routines not directly related to breast-feeding will contribute to its successful initiation by increasing a woman's sense of security, preventing unnecessary discomfort and ensuring maximum moral support during labour and delivery.

Influencing the influential

The content of training programmes in paediatrics, obstetrics and
public health and the attitudes of teaching staff have a direct influence on breast-feeding policies and programmes in health services. Health workers within these services are in turn well placed
to cooperate directly with health decision-makers in identifying
aspects of their programmes for maternal and child care that help
or hinder breast-feeding and in deciding how to make im-
provements. Related policy decisions concern the structure and
functioning of health services (as discussed on page 11) as much
as the content of training curricula for health personnel; both are
fundamental in determining how services can protect, promote
and support breast-feeding.

Health workers, particularly through their professional associa-
tions, are well placed to act as sources of authoritative information on breast-feeding, to serve as forums for reviewing related
policies and programmes, and to promote appropriate action in-
side and outside the health sector.

4. Procedures and individual care

Prenatal care: history, physical examination and counselling

All pregnant women and mothers should benefit from educational and promotional activities relating to breast-feeding. The key to counselling women on breast-feeding is to tailor a personal approach to specific needs identified from knowledge of both the individual and her social environment. If a consulting woman is multiparous, has successfully breast-fed a previous child or children, comes from a society where breast-feeding is common and intends to breast-feed her next child, it is unlikely that a health worker will face any particular promotional or educational difficulties. If, on the other hand, a woman is a primipara from a society where bottle-feeding is the norm, the health worker should not underestimate the difficulties associated with guiding and supporting even someone who has expressed a desire to breast-feed.

From a health worker's first contact with a pregnant woman, and as part of her health history, careful assessment should be made of attitudes, beliefs, knowledge and experience in relation to infant feeding. The history should also provide information on her social circumstances and dietary habits and practices and those of her family, including usual food intake, preferences, dislikes and taboos. This information can be used later to evaluate a woman's nutritional status and to advise her on an appropriate diet during pregnancy and lactation (see next section). It will also form the basis for future education and support in relation to breast-feeding.

During a woman's physical examination, her breasts should be checked for any anatomical malformation that could interfere with breast-feeding, for example inverted nipples. This condition is rare and mild cases may be treated in the antenatal clinic. Simple exercises performed by the woman during the last trimester of pregnancy can help to prepare her nipples for successful breast-feeding. Women with small breasts should be reassured that size has little relation to lactation performance.

Every expectant mother should be provided with information on infant feeding that has been adapted to suit her personal history and socioeconomic circumstances and that emphasizes the advantages of breast-feeding. The help provided by experienced mothers individually, members of mothers' support groups collectively, or breast-feeding counsellors can be extremely effective in this connection. Group sessions organized to meet the health education needs of mothers-to-be should have breast-feeding among their priority health and nutrition messages. These sessions should complement, rather than replace, the individual attention given to women by doctors, midwives, nurses and breast-feeding counsellors.

Suggested action

A woman's health history provides a basis for understanding her disposition towards breast-feeding, and health workers should counsel women on breast-feeding in the light of knowledge of both the individual and her social environment. Educational and instructional material should be prepared and adapted to ensure that every expectant mother is fully informed of the health and nutritional benefits of breast-feeding and techniques to ensure its successful initiation and establishment.

Prenatal care: advice on dietary intake and use of drugs

Nutritional status during pregnancy is extremely important. Not only does dietary intake influence pregnancy outcome for both mother and child, but it also has a direct impact on future lactation performance. The nutritional requirements of pregnant women are increased in comparison with those of non-pregnant women, although not by as much as once believed. During pregnancy, a number of metabolic and functional adaptations occur, particularly in mechanisms for energy utilization. While the notion that a pregnant woman should "eat for two" might be a useful educational analogy in cases where dietary intake needs to be increased, it is nevertheless an exaggeration. Healthy well-nourished mothers can go through pregnancy without a significant increase in their dietary intake.

A pregnant woman's energy intake should be adjusted to take into account her nutritional status and level of physical activity. Women who are required to maintain high rates of activity, particularly if they are undernourished, should be encouraged to increase their energy intake. Ideally, they should be provided with dietary supplements. Well-nourished women, on the other hand, should be advised not to increase their normal energy intake to avoid gaining too much weight. The amount and rate of weight increase during pregnancy are generally a good guide for making individual recommendations on energy intake.

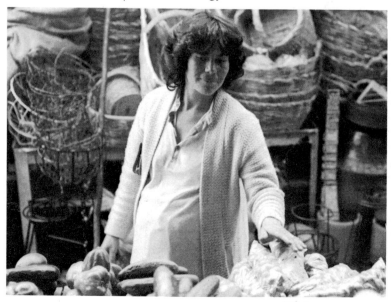

WHO/T. Kelly (19776)

15

It is now recognized that adequate energy intake is important throughout pregnancy and not only, as was once believed, during late pregnancy when the nutritional requirements of the fetus are greatest. Where necessary, therefore, energy intake should be increased at the beginning of pregnancy, given the need to build up the fat reserves required later, including for lactation, when energy needs are particularly high.

In well-nourished populations in developed countries, the weight gain during pregnancy is about 12.5 kg. Women of small stature tend to have smaller babies and would logically fall in the lower range of normal weight gains and hence need less additional energy than the average. Obese women need to gain less fat than slimmer women, and women who are underweight for their height need to gain more than the average.

Special attention should be given to the overall composition of a pregnant woman's diet, which should be mixed and varied to ensure an adequate intake of protein, vitamins and other essential nutrients. Cultural taboos notwithstanding, there is generally no need to avoid any specific foods during pregnancy.

It is also extremely important to detect and correct any specific nutrient deficiencies, for example conditions related to an insufficient dietary intake of iron, iodine or vitamin A. These conditions present added risks for infants, which should be taken into account when recommendations are made on dietary intake and supplementation for pregnant women.

As regards nutrition education in general, formal group sessions may be useful for imparting information on such topics as the advantages of breast-feeding, the nutritional value of breast milk, breast-feeding techniques, and general dietary principles during pregnancy and lactation. Once again, however, emphasis should be placed on individual counselling.

The use of alcohol, tobacco, excessive amounts of caffeine, and other drugs may be particularly harmful during pregnancy because of their effect on the fetus. Smoking, for example, is associated with low birth weight, while the use of alcohol and other "recreational" drugs has been linked to dysfunction of the nervous system and other congenital defects. Mothers-to-be should be made aware of these problems and encouraged to avoid using such drugs during pregnancy.

Likewise, some medicinal drugs may traverse the placenta and have adverse consequences for the fetus. Women should avoid unnecessary medication during pregnancy and lactation, and health personnel who prescribe medicaments should familiarize themselves with their possible undesirable effects on the fetus and infant. Nevertheless, depending on individual need, it may be necessary to provide some women with specific therapy, for example iron tablets to control anaemia or chemoprophylaxis against malaria. Particular caution should be taken with new drugs that have not yet been fully tested.

Suggested action

An adequate maternal diet should be ensured by various means, including the provision of appropriate health and nutrition education for women. Women should be discouraged from using alcohol, tobacco, excessive caffeine, and other non-medicinal drugs during pregnancy and lactation; they should also avoid unnecessary medication.

Care for the mother during and immediately after delivery

Many delivery and perinatal care routines, which are often characterized by their "surgical" and "aseptic" approach, were originally established to control perinatal infections or to facilitate the work of doctors and other hospital staff. While not all of these routines impair mother–child bonding, their effect on lactation performance is frequently negative.

A woman's experience during labour and delivery affects her motivation towards breast-feeding and the ease with which she initiates it. The sensitivity and responsiveness of the health staff to her needs, including respect for her dignity and privacy, contribute to her comfort and sense of ease. To reduce the discomfort of labour to a minimum, a woman should be allowed to move around, adopt the most comfortable position, and have a loved one or other person of confidence to accompany and support her. Such simple practices can reduce the duration of labour and the need for oxytocin, surgical interventions and sedatives, as well as improve prospects for successful breast-feeding.

The need for sedatives, analgesics and anaesthetics should be carefully considered. While it is important to reduce a woman's physical discomfort, the indiscriminate or excessive use of such medicaments may well reduce her ability to have a normal delivery, induce drowsiness, prevent her establishing close contact with her infant immediately after delivery, and diminish the newborn infant's sucking capabilities. Care should also be taken to avoid administering any medicaments, including hormones, that could directly interfere with the initiation and establishment of breast-feeding.

The infant's rooting and sucking reflexes are particularly strong immediately after normal delivery, and a mother is usually keen to see and touch her child. Encouraging skin-to-skin contact between mother and infant immediately after birth and permitting the infant to suck at the breast will be beneficial, and will help to strengthen initial mother–child bonding and stimulate breast-milk secretion. The infant's sucking movements will also stimulate the release of oxytocin, which facilitates the expulsion of the placenta and uterine contraction during the third stage of labour.

A mother's need for rest after delivery can be satisfied later; in fact, rest will be facilitated by initial close contact with her infant during the first half-hour or so. The newborn infant should therefore be cleaned and dried — a bath is not necessary — and placed over the mother's abdomen for her to take and put to her breast. The routine application of silver nitrate or antibiotic eye drops to prevent conjunctivitis may be delayed for 15 minutes or so in order not to interfere with eye-to-eye contact between mother and child. The infant should remain close to the mother while in the delivery room.

It is obvious that such practices are not possible in the case of a caesarean section or other major surgical intervention. Nevertheless, the principle of allowing close mother–child contact as soon as possible after birth remains unchanged.

Care of the newborn infant

The care of the infant during the first 2 or 3 days of life and, in particular, how the infant is fed have a very strong influence on a mother's breast-feeding performance.

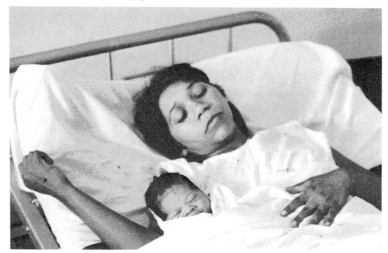

WHO/P. Abensur (20569)

19

The infant's birth weight should be entered on a growth chart, which will serve as an important reference point for both mother and health worker for purposes of follow-up care.

Rooming-in

The skin-to-skin and eye-to-eye contact between mother and child that was established immediately after birth should be maintained, and a mother should have unlimited access to her child. Rooming-in should therefore replace the practice of keeping mother and child in separate rooms and permitting "visits" only according to schedule. Rooming-in has a number of important advantages over separating infants from their mothers. For example, it facilitates bonding, permits breast-feeding on demand and allows for closer contact with the father and other family members.

The risk of neonatal infection, which is a major concern, is in fact lower in the mother's room than in the closed environment of a nursery, where serious epidemics can occur. Maintaining the mother–infant contact that was established immediately after birth favours the colonization of the infant's skin and gastrointestinal tract with the mother's microorganisms, which tend to be non-pathogenic and against which she has antibodies in her breast milk. The infant is thus simultaneously exposed to, and protected against, the organisms for which active immunity will be developed only later in life.

In contrast, infants kept in nurseries tend to be exposed to the bacteria of the hospital staff — microorganisms which, on the whole, are more pathogenic and often resistant to many antimicrobial drugs, and for which breast milk contains no specific antibodies. This explains the ease with which epidemics of skin, respiratory and gastrointestinal infections develop in such environments. Rooming-in also eliminates the need for staff to transport infants to and from their mothers' rooms, occasionally over long distances within the hospital or clinic, and thus increases staff availability for other tasks.

There are a number of ways to organize rooming-in, according to the layout of the particular maternity ward or hospital. The operative principle is to allow a mother free and easy access to her infant through close proximity, whether the infant shares the mother's bed, which offers several important advantages, or is in another bed in the same room.

Feeding

The infant should be permitted to suck freely at the breast, frequently and without any fixed timetable. This will ensure that the infant has the full benefit of colostrum, which is extremely important immunologically (to prevent common diseases), nutritionally (to provide vitamins and minerals) and developmentally (to ensure maturation of the intestinal mucosa).

Frequent sucking and emptying of the breasts will also favour better and faster establishment of lactation. Strong sucking is a potent stimulus for the secretion of prolactin and oxytocin, which respectively initiate milk secretion and stimulate the let-down reflex that makes breast milk available to the infant, in addition to accelerating postpartum uterine contraction and involution. The correct positioning of the infant at the breast is important so that enough of the breast is taken into the month to ensure sufficient milk supply and efficient milk transfer; in addition, it facilitates feeding and helps prevent sore or cracked nipples and breast engorgement.

Exclusive breast-feeding should be the norm. Infants should usually be given nothing orally but breast milk during their stay in the hospital or clinic. The administration by bottle and teat of water, herbal teas, glucose solutions or, worse still, milk-based formulas not only is unnecessary on nutritional grounds, but reduces the infant's sucking capacity and therefore the mother's lactation stimulus. Furthermore, such practices increase the risk of introducing infection and, in the case of milk-based formulas, of sensitizing an infant to cow's-milk proteins.

Under normal conditions, natural energy and water reserves are sufficient to sustain the newborn for the first few days of life while lactation is being fully established. Keeping the newborn in a warm and not excessively dry environment is therefore recommended to prevent unnecessary energy losses due to cold, or water losses through perspiration.

Only small quantities of breast-milk substitutes are ordinarily required in health care facilities for the few infants who cannot be breast-fed. Their provision to the infants in question should not interfere with the promotion of breast-feeding for the great majority.

Suggested action

The birth weight of every infant should be entered on a growth chart. Rooming-in should be the norm for all healthy newborn infants, and mothers should be encouraged to feed their infants on demand. Exclusive breast-feeding should be promoted, and infants should not be provided with any other food or drink unless medically indicated.

Discharge and follow-up care

The fact that so many infants currently leave hospitals and clinics already bottle-fed is contributing considerably to the decline in the prevalence of breast-feeding. Bottle-feeding may be introduced with the best of intentions, and may even be considered a temporary measure until lactation is firmly established. In fact, it serves as a potent force against the successful initiation and maintenance of lactation by reducing the frequency and strength of sucking by the infant. Often, the result is that mothers are encouraged to continue the artificial feeding mode begun in the health care institution.

General advice

Mothers should be informed that alternating between an artificial stimulus (rubber teat) and a natural stimulus (the breast) only confuses their infants' oral response. Since less work is required to suck at a rubber teat, cheek muscles weaken and the desire for the breast is lost. To avoid any decline in milk production due to poor sucking, neither artificial teats nor pacifiers (also called dummies or soothers) should be given to breast-feeding infants.

In the rare cases when complementary feeding is necessary, food can be provided by teaspoon, dropper or small cup.

The amount of time that mothers and infants remain in hospitals or clinics following normal delivery varies greatly — as little as 12–24 hours in some cases and as much as 2–3 days or even a week in others. Lactation is usually not yet well established, and might not even have started, by the time a mother and child are discharged. It is thus important that the mother leaves the hospital or clinic clear and confident about what she should do to breast-feed successfully. If the mother is inexperienced, she should be informed about the milk let-down reflex and the mechanics of lactation and instructed in breast-feeding techniques. She should be advised how to care for her breasts and to avoid excessive washing, which may lead to sore or cracked nipples. She should also be encouraged to feed her infant on demand and not to give anything other than breast milk. Finally, in cases where breast-feeding is temporarily delayed or interrupted for any reason, or when a mother is separated from her infant, she should be shown how to initiate or maintain lactation by other means.

In many countries, women have established social support groups to help mothers who wish to breast-feed their children. Health workers should support the creation and functioning of such groups, and refer mothers, particularly those who are young and inexperienced, to them when they are discharged from the hospital or clinic. The individual counselling and the health education and information materials provided by such groups can serve as an important adjunct to the efforts of health workers. The distribution of such materials should be encouraged within the health system.

Nutritional requirements during lactation

Nutritional requirements during lactation are greater than during pregnancy. If a mother was well nourished during pregnancy, she will have adequate energy reserves in the form of fat that can be used to compensate partially for her additional requirements. The use of this fat, combined with the loss of the water that accumulated during pregnancy and absorption of uterine tissue, will

23

result in weight loss during the weeks immediately following delivery. Mothers should be instructed about the need for an adequate diet in order to sustain lactation without depleting their own nutrient stores. Particular attention should be given to intake of protein, calcium and vitamins.

If the dietary energy recommendations for pregnancy have been met, the average additional energy requirement during the first 6 months of lactation is about 2090 kJ/day. Allowances during this and subsequent periods will need to be adjusted according to maternal fat stores and patterns of activity. For example, to prevent any further deterioration in nutritional status, a greater increase in dietary intake is required for an undernourished woman who has not gained adequate weight during pregnancy, and therefore has insufficient fat reserves at the beginning of lactation.

Discharge

In some countries it is a common practice in maternity services to provide mothers, on discharge, with a variety of baby- and personal-care products that have been supplied free of charge by commercial enterprises. The competent authorities should ensure that such "discharge packs" contain nothing that might interfere with the successful initiation and establishment of breast-feeding, for example feeding bottles and teats, pacifiers and infant formula.

The mothers or other family members, as appropriate, of infants who are not fed on breast milk should receive adequate instructions for the correct preparation and feeding of breast-milk substitutes, and a warning against the health hazards of incorrect preparation. However, such instructions should not be provided in the presence of breast-feeding mothers.

Follow-up care

An extremely useful, and in some health services routine, practice is a home visit by a health worker a week or so after discharge to see how mother and child are getting on, answer questions and generally help with any problems that may have arisen. In any case,

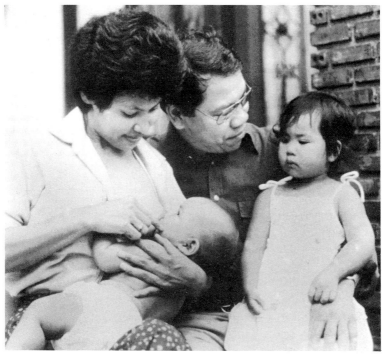

at the time of discharge a mother should be given an appointment
for her first follow-up visit for postnatal and infant care, in addition
to being informed how to deal with problems that may arise, such as
sore nipples and an infant's sucking difficulties. Health workers
should be prepared to take appropriate action to resolve these
and other problems and to answer any questions a mother
may have.

Mothers occasionally have doubts about the quantity and quality
of their milk. If they were to begin giving other foods to complement their breast milk, the probable result would be an early inter-
ruption of lactation. It is therefore important to reassure mothers
by periodically examining their children, whose health status and
growth should provide the most convincing evidence of the
nutritional adequacy of breast milk. Follow-up of infants by the
health services including periodic weighing and growth

25

monitoring is indispensable; the growth chart, where the infant's birth weight has been entered as the obvious point of departure, is ideal for this purpose. Follow-up visits also provide an opportunity to give mothers practical tips about breast-feeding and ensure that all other maternal and child health services, particularly immunization and family planning, are provided in an appropriate and timely fashion.

Suggested action

By the time of their discharge from the hospital or clinic, mothers should be appropriately briefed on the physiology and mechanics of lactation so that they are confident about how to breast-feed; they should be informed of the existence of social support groups, if any, to help them with breast-feeding and be referred to these groups if appropriate; they should be advised on nutritional requirements during lactation; and appointments should be made for follow-up visits for them and their infants.

5. Conclusion

In every country, the competent authorities should implement the health and social measures required to protect, promote and support breast-feeding. They should ensure that the most appropriate choice with regard to infant feeding is made within families, and that the health system supports this decision in every way. This implies that mothers are adequately informed about matters relating to infant feeding, receive appropriate family and community support to facilitate and encourage breast-feeding, and are protected from influences that inhibit it. In particular, every effort should be made to protect, promote and support breast-feeding in and through the health services.

This statement and its annex can serve as a guide to the kinds of practical steps that should be taken by maternity services in this regard. The competent authorities in countries are invited to adapt it to suit local health and socioeconomic circumstances so as to encourage and facilitate the initiation and establishment of breast-feeding by the mothers in their care.

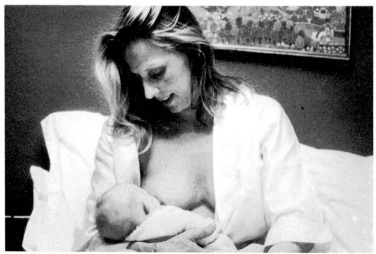

WHO/J.-F. Chrétien (C-873)

Annex

Check-list for evaluating the adequacy of support for breast-feeding in maternity hospitals, wards and clinics[1]

The following check-list has been prepared for use by the competent authorities in countries — health and nutrition policy-makers; managers of maternal and child health and family planning services; clinicians, midwives, nursing personnel and other support staff in maternity services and facilities for the care of newborn infants; health workers' organizations; and mothers' support groups. It is intended to be a suggestive rather than exhaustive inventory of the kinds of practical steps that can be taken within and through maternity services to protect, promote and support breast-feeding, and should be used in conjunction with the main text of the joint WHO/UNICEF statement. Under ideal circumstances, the answer to all of the questions in the check-list will be "Yes". A negative reply may indicate an inappropriate practice or routine that should be modified in accordance with the statement.

---

[1] Hereinafter collectively referred to as "health care facilities".

Policy

1. Does the health care facility have an explicit policy for protecting, promoting and supporting breast-feeding?
2. Is this policy communicated to those responsible for managing and providing maternity services (for example in oral briefings when new staff are employed; in manuals, guidelines and other written materials; or by supervisory personnel)?
3. Is there a mechanism for evaluating the effectiveness of the breast-feeding policy? For example:
   - Are data collected on the prevalence of breast-feeding initiation and breast-feeding at the time of discharge of mothers and their infants from the health care facility?
   - Is there a system for assessing related health care practices and training and promotional materials, including those commonly used by antenatal and postnatal services?
4. Are the cooperation and support of all interested parties, particularly health care providers, breast-feeding counsellors and mothers' support groups, but also the general public, sought in developing and implementing the health care facility's breast-feeding policy?

Staff training

5. Are all health care staff well aware of the importance and advantages of breast-feeding and acquainted with the health care facility's policy and services to protect, promote and support breast-feeding?
6. Has the health care facility provided specialized training in lactation management to specific staff members?

Structure and functioning of services

7. Do antenatal records indicate whether breast-feeding has been discussed with a pregnant woman? Is it noted:
   - Whether a woman has indicated her intention to breast-feed?
   - Whether her breasts have been examined?

- Whether her breast-feeding history has been taken?
- How long and how often she has already breast-fed?
- Whether she previously encountered any problems and, if so, what kind?
- What type of help she received, if any, and from whom?

8. Is a mother's antenatal record available at the time of delivery?
   - If not, is the information in point 7 nevertheless communicated to the staff of the health care facility?
   - Does a woman who has never breast-fed, or who has previously encountered problems with breast-feeding, receive special attention and support from the staff of the health care facility?

9. Does the health care facility take into account a woman's intention to breast-feed when deciding on the use of a sedative, an analgesic or an anaesthetic, if any, during labour and delivery?
   - Are staff familiar with the effects of such medicaments on breast-feeding?

10. In general, are newborn infants:
    - Shown to their mothers within 5 minutes after completion of the second stage of labour?
    - Shown/given to their mothers before silver nitrate or antibiotic drops are administered prophylactically to the infants' eyes?
    - Given to their mothers to hold and put to the breast within a half-hour of completion of the second stage of labour, and allowed to remain with them for at least one hour?

11. Does the health care facility have a rooming-in policy? That is, do infants remain with their mothers throughout their stay?
    - Are mothers allowed to have their infants with them in their beds?
    - If the infants stay in cots, are these placed close to the mothers' beds?
    - If rooming-in applies only during daytime hours, are infants at least brought frequently (every 3–4 hours) to their mothers at night?

12. Is it the health care facility's policy to restrict the giving of prelacteal feeds, that is any food or drink other than breast milk, before breast-feeding has been established?

Health education

13. Are all expectant mothers advised on nutritional requirements during pregnancy and lactation, and on the dangers associated with the use of drugs?
14. Are information and education on breast-feeding routinely provided to pregnant women during antenatal care?
15. Are staff members or counsellors who have specialized training in lactation management available full time to advise breast-feeding mothers during their stay in the health care facility and in preparation for their discharge? Are mothers informed:
    - About the physiology of lactation and how to maintain it?
    - How to prevent and manage common problems like breast engorgement and sore or cracked nipples?
    - Where to turn, for example to breast-feeding support groups, to deal with these or related problems? (Do breast-feeding support groups have access to the health care facility?)
16. Are support and counselling on how to initiate and maintain breast-feeding routinely provided for women who:
    - Have undergone caesarean section?
    - Have delivered prematurely?
    - Have delivered low-birth-weight infants?
    - Have infants who are in special care for any reason?
17. Are breast-feeding mothers provided with printed materials that give relevant guidance and information?

Discharge

18. If "discharge packs" containing baby- and personal-care products are provided to mothers when they leave the hospital or clinic, is it the policy of the health care facility to ensure that they contain nothing that might interfere with the successful initiation and establishment of breast-feeding, for example feeding bottles and teats, pacifiers and infant formula?
19. Are mothers or other family members, as appropriate, of infants who are not fed on breast milk given adequate instruc-

tions for the correct preparation and feeding of breast-milk substitutes, and a warning against the health hazards of incorrect preparation?

- Is it the policy of the health care facility not to give such instructions in the presence of breast-feeding mothers?

20. Is every mother given an appointment for her first follow-up visit for postnatal and infant care?

- Is she informed how to deal with any problems that may arise meanwhile in relation to breast-feeding?